Thriving with Type 2:

Insider Tips for Living Well with Diabetes

By

John Poe

Copyright © by John Poe 2024.

All rights reserved.

Before this document is duplicated or reproduced in any manner, the publisher's consent must be gained. Therefore, the contents within can neither be stored electronically, transferred, or kept in a database. Neither in Part nor full can the document be copied, scanned, faxed, or retained without approval from the publisher or creator.

Table Of Contents

Introduction

Greetings and welcome to "Thriving with Type 2: Insider Tips for Leading a Healthy Lifestyle with Diabetes."

Together, we'll explore doable tactics, insider knowledge, and empowering guidance for controlling type 2 diabetes and improving your general well-being in these pages.

Although managing type 2 diabetes might be difficult, it's crucial to keep in mind that success is achievable with the correct information, resources, and attitude. This book is meant to be your travel companion, providing you with advice and insights from professionals and others who have been there before you.

We lay the groundwork for the book's contents in this introduction. We'll talk about the aims and objectives of "Thriving with Type 2," give you a rundown of what to expect, and offer a message of empowerment and hope to people who are dealing with type 2 diabetes.

The Book's Goals

"Thriving with Type 2" aims to empower people with type 2 diabetes to take charge of their health, adopt self-care routines, and live their best lives despite the difficulties associated with managing a chronic illness. We think that having diabetes may be successfully managed, along with thriving and leading a happy life, if one has the appropriate information, resources, and assistance.

How Things Are Anticipated

We'll explore a wide range of subjects connected to living well with type 2 diabetes in the ensuing chapters. Each chapter is jam-packed with useful guidance, doable suggestions, and insider knowledge to help you navigate the difficulties of managing diabetes with confidence and ease. These range from comprehending the illness and creating a support system to managing nutrition, physical activity, medication, and more.

A Word of Inspiration and Strength
It can be difficult to manage type 2 diabetes at times, but it's crucial to keep in mind that you are not by yourself. You have access to an extensive network of resources, such as this book, internet communities, support groups,

and medical professionals. You can overcome challenges, accomplish your goals, and thrive with type 2 diabetes by educating yourself, getting help when you need it, and adopting a proactive approach.

Remember that you are capable, strong, and worthy of a happy, healthy life as you set out on this adventure with us. Together, let's explore the methods, approaches, and understandings that will enable you to flourish in the face of type 2 diabetes and greet every day with vigor and confidence.

Chapter One

An understanding of diabetes type two

We explore the foundations of type 2 diabetes in this chapter of "Thriving with Type 2," including crucial information on the illness's causes, symptoms, and effects on general health and wellbeing.

Describe Type 2 Diabetes.

High blood sugar (glucose) levels are a hallmark of type 2 diabetes, a chronic metabolic disease. Type 2 diabetes usually occurs when the body becomes resistant to insulin or is unable to produce enough insulin to maintain normal blood sugar levels. Type 1 diabetes is caused by an immune system attack on the pancreatic cells that make insulin.

Factors at Risk and Their Causes

Type 2 diabetes is a result of a combination of environmental, lifestyle, and genetic factors. Type 2 diabetes can be greatly increased by lifestyle factors such as poor food, lack of physical activity, obesity, and smoking, even if some people may be genetically predisposed to the disease. Additional risk factors encompass age, race, a family history of diabetes, and specific medical disorders including polycystic ovarian syndrome (PCOS) and high blood pressure.

Signs and the Prognosis

Type 2 diabetes symptoms might vary from person to person and may appear gradually over time. Increased thirst, frequent urination, unexpected weight loss, exhaustion, hazy eyesight, sluggish wound healing, and recurrent infections are typical symptoms. On the other hand, some people do not exhibit any symptoms at all or just have minor ones that go unnoticed for years.

Blood tests that evaluate hemoglobin A1c (HbA1c) levels, oral glucose tolerance, or fasting blood glucose levels are commonly used to diagnose type 2 diabetes. When blood glucose levels are regularly higher than normal ranges, a diagnosis is verified.

Consequences for Health and Wellness

Numerous acute and long-term consequences, such as cardiovascular disease, neuropathy (nerve damage), nephropathy (kidney damage), retinopathy (eye damage), foot ulcers, and amputations, can result from untreated or inadequately managed type 2 diabetes. Nonetheless, many of these issues can be avoided or postponed with appropriate management and lifestyle changes, enabling people with type 2 diabetes to have long, healthy lives.

In the following chapters of "Thriving with Type 2," we'll delve into professional advice and doable tactics for successfully managing type 2 diabetes, including dietary recommendations, exercise regimens, drug schedules, and more. You may

take charge of your health and manage
type 2 diabetes by being aware of its
intricacies and taking an active attitude
to self-care.

Chapter Two

Putting Up a Support Network

We discuss the value of creating a solid support network in this chapter of "Thriving with Type 2" to help you deal with the difficulties of having diabetes. A network of support can play a major role in properly managing diabetes and enhancing overall well-being. This support can come from peers in the diabetic community, family, friends, and healthcare professionals.

Support Types

Family and friends: They can help with diabetes management by offering emotional support, motivation, and helpful advice. They can help you plan meals and get exercise, they can be there to listen, and they can go with you to doctor's appointments.

Healthcare Team: The doctors, nurses, dietitians, and diabetes educators that make up your healthcare team are essential to the management of diabetes. To assist you deal with the challenges of diabetes care, they can offer professional advice, personalized treatment regimens, and continuing support.

Support Groups: You can meet people who comprehend the difficulties of living with diabetes by joining an online community or diabetic support group. A secure place to talk about experiences, get guidance, and get support from others going through similar things is provided via support groups.

Diabetes Educators: Medical professionals with training in diabetes management, and certified diabetes educators (CDEs) can offer individualized guidance, counseling, and support. They can help you build skills for self-care and illness management, as well as provide helpful advice and answers to your queries.

Some Advice for Creating a Support Network

Communicate Your Needs: Tell your loved ones and the medical staff exactly what you need, want, and are concerned about when it comes to managing your diabetes. To establish trust and make sure you get the help you need, effective communication is crucial.

Look for Resources: Make use of all the resources at your disposal, such as books, websites, chat rooms, support groups, and local initiatives. You can get important information, direction, and support from these resources to help you deal with the difficulties of having diabetes.

Establish Boundaries: Setting limits and giving self-care priority is crucial, even while assistance from others is priceless. Don't be afraid to ask for assistance when you need it, and be upfront about your requirements and limitations. Recall that if you're feeling overburdened or need some alone time, it's acceptable to say no.

Express gratitude: Let others know how much you appreciate the help you get from your family, your medical team, and other members of your support network. Gratitude creates good relationships and tightens the connections within your support system.

You can feel empowered, motivated, and better prepared to manage diabetes and enhance your overall quality of life by creating a support network that consists of friends, family, medical experts, and peers in the diabetic community. We'll go deeper into doable tactics and knowledgeable advice for controlling diabetes and improving well-being with the help of your network in the upcoming chapters of "Thriving with Type 2."

Chapter Three

Dietary Guidelines and Meal Scheduling

We examine the vital role that nutrition plays in successfully controlling type 2 diabetes in this chapter of "Thriving with Type 2." Controlling blood sugar levels, managing weight, and lowering the risk of complications from diabetes can all be achieved by choosing healthy foods and adhering to a balanced diet plan.

Nutrition's Significance

Blood Sugar Control: Blood sugar levels can be stabilized and daytime spikes and crashes can be avoided by eating the proper meals in moderation and managing portion amounts.

Weight management: Maintaining or losing weight is aided by a nutritious diet, and this is crucial for reducing insulin resistance and enhancing general health.

Heart Health: Lowering the risk of cardiovascular problems, like heart disease and stroke, which are more common in people with type 2 diabetes, can be achieved by eating a heart-healthy diet.

Important Elements of a Diabetes-Friendly Diet

carbs: Choose complex carbs over refined ones. These include whole grains, fruits, vegetables, and legumes. Complex carbohydrates are higher in fiber and minerals and have less of an effect on blood sugar levels.

Proteins: To help stabilize blood sugar levels and encourage fullness, choose lean protein sources such as fish, chicken, tofu, beans, and lentils.

Fats: Limit trans and saturated fats, which are included in processed and fried meals, and choose heart-healthy fats like those in avocados, nuts, seeds, and olive oil.

Portion Control: Be mindful of serving sizes to limit calorie intake and prevent overindulging. When in doubt, estimate portion amounts using measuring cups, food scales, or visual cues.

Useful Advice for Meal Planning

Assemble a Balanced Plate: Try to put non-starchy veggies on half of it, lean protein on one quarter, and whole grains or starchy vegetables on the other quarter.

Plan: Give yourself enough time to organize your meals and snacks in advance, taking into account things like the amount of carbohydrates in each meal and the timing of them.

Read Food Labels: Acquire the skill of reading food labels to spot hidden sugars, carbs, and bad fats in prepared foods. Seek for products with the least amount of added sugar and processing.

Add variation: To make sure you're getting a wide range of nutrients and flavors, add variation to your diet by consuming a variety of meals. To make meals engaging and pleasurable, try experimenting with various cuisines, flavors, and cooking methods.

Keep Yourself Hydrated: To stay hydrated and promote general health, sip lots of water throughout the day. Water, herbal tea, or infused water are better options than sugar-filled beverages.

Individuals with type 2 diabetes can effectively manage their illness, maintain blood sugar levels, and enhance their overall health and well-being by prioritizing nutrition and meal planning. We'll go deeper into doable tactics and professional advice for implementing a balanced diet into your daily routine in the upcoming chapters of "Thriving with Type 2."

Chapter Four

Exercise and Physical Activity

We discuss the value of exercise and physical activity in properly controlling type 2 diabetes in this chapter of "Thriving with Type 2." Frequent exercise aids weight management, cardiovascular health, and overall well-being in addition to helping lower blood sugar levels.

Advantages of Exercise

Blood Sugar Control: Exercise lowers blood sugar levels and lowers the risk of problems from diabetes by assisting your body in using insulin more effectively.

Weight management: Maintaining a healthy weight and body fat percentage is crucial for reducing insulin resistance and enhancing general health.

Heart Health: Cardiovascular issues like heart disease and stroke are less likely in people with type 2 diabetes because exercise strengthens the heart and increases circulation.

Different Forms of Exercise

Aerobic Exercise: Exercises like walking, jogging, cycling, swimming, dancing, and aerobics that raise heart rate and respiration are great for enhancing blood sugar regulation and cardiovascular health.

Strength Training: Including resistance training activities in your workout routine, such as bodyweight exercises, resistance band exercises, and weightlifting, will help you gain muscle mass, increase your insulin sensitivity, and manage your weight.

Exercises for Flexibility and Balance: Yoga, tai chi, and stretching can increase mobility, flexibility, and balance. These benefits lower the risk of falls and accidents while also enhancing general well-being.

How to Begin an Exercise Programme

See Your Healthcare Provider: It's Important to See Your Healthcare Provider Before Beginning Any Exercise Programme, Particularly if You Have Any Underlying Health Conditions or Concerns.

Establish Realistic Goals: As your fitness level increases, progressively raise the intensity, duration, and frequency of your workouts. Begin with small, attainable goals.

Discover Interest-Based Activities: Select pastimes that suit your interests, way of life, and physical capabilities. Exercise should be pleasurable, whether it's through sports, dancing to your favorite music, or taking walks in the outdoors.

Develop the Habit: Incorporate regular workouts into your weekly schedule and view them as unchangeable appointments. To fully benefit from physical activity, consistency is essential.

How to Exercise Safely
Monitor Blood Sugar Levels: If you take insulin or other medications that can lower blood sugar levels, be sure to

check your blood sugar levels before, during, and after exercise.

Keep Hydrated: To stay hydrated and promote peak performance, drink lots of water before, during, and after exercise.

Pay Attention to Your Body: While exercising, pay attention to how you're feeling and change the duration or intensity as necessary. If you feel lightheaded, dizzy, have chest pain, or any other unsettling symptoms, stop exercising.

Including regular exercise and physical activity in your routine can help you better control your blood sugar, strengthen your cardiovascular system, and feel better overall. The upcoming chapters of "Thriving with Type 2" will go into further detail on doable tactics and professional advice for fitting exercise into your daily routine and getting beyond typical obstacles.

Chapter Five

Medication Administration

In "Thriving with Type 2," we explore the critical facets of type 2 diabetes medication management in this chapter. Although dietary and activity changes are important parts of managing diabetes, medications are frequently required to help control blood sugar levels and avoid complications.

Diabetes Medication Types

Oral Drugs: A variety of classes of oral drugs are available to treat type 2 diabetes, such as:

Metformin is a frequently prescribed drug that lowers blood sugar levels by enhancing insulin sensitivity and decreasing the liver's synthesis of glucose.

Sulfonylureas: Induce increased insulin production by the pancreas.

DPP-4 inhibitors: Promote insulin synthesis and decrease glucose synthesis in the liver to help lower blood sugar levels.

SGLT2 inhibitors: Cause the kidneys to excrete glucose from the bloodstream through urine, lowering blood sugar levels.

GLP-1 receptor agonists: Decrease glucose synthesis and increase insulin synthesis in the liver, slow down digestion, and decrease hunger.
Injectable Drugs: To properly control blood sugar levels, some people with type 2 diabetes may require injectable drugs such as insulin or GLP-1 receptor agonists.

Things to Take Account of When Managing Medication

Effectiveness: Based on your unique needs, preferences, and health state, work with your healthcare professional to choose the right medicine or combination of medications.

Side Effects: Recognise the possible negative effects of diabetic drugs and instantly report any worries or unfavorable reactions to your healthcare professional.

Adherence: To obtain the best blood sugar management, it's critical to take your medications as directed and follow the suggested dosages and timings.

Monitoring: To make sure that your medications are successfully managing your diabetes, check your blood sugar levels regularly as instructed by your healthcare professional.

Combining Lifestyle Changes with Medication Management

Complementary Approach: Rather than taking the place of dietary changes, physical activity, and weight control, medication treatment should support these lifestyle adjustments.

Monitoring Blood Sugar Levels: Check your blood sugar levels frequently to determine how well your medications are working and to make any necessary modifications with your healthcare practitioner.

Healthy behaviors: To support general well-being and improve the efficacy of your drugs, keep putting a high priority on healthy behaviors like a balanced diet, frequent exercise, stress reduction, and enough sleep.

Collaboration with Healthcare Team: Keep lines of communication open with your diabetes care team and healthcare provider to make sure that your prescriptions are in line with your treatment objectives and that they are modified as needed to account for changes in your lifestyle or health.

You can achieve optimal blood sugar control, lower your risk of complications, and enhance your overall quality of life with type 2 diabetes by managing your medications well in addition to making lifestyle improvements. The upcoming chapters of "Thriving with Type 2" will go into greater detail on doable tactics and professional advice for managing medications and enhancing diabetic treatment.

Chapter Six

Monitoring Blood Sugar and Practicing Self-Care

This chapter of "Thriving with Type 2" delves into the significance of self-care routines and blood sugar monitoring for the successful management of type 2 diabetes. Self-care routines and routine blood sugar testing can help people with diabetes maintain control over their illness, avoid complications, and enhance their general well-being.

The Significance of Monitoring Blood Sugar

Blood Sugar Control: By keeping an eye on blood sugar levels, people can assess how effectively they are controlling their diabetes and modify their treatment plan as necessary.

Finding Patterns: Consistent blood sugar monitoring can assist spot trends and patterns, including spikes or dips, in blood sugar levels. This information can then be used to guide dietary decisions, medication adjustments, and lifestyle changes.

Prevention of Complications: People with diabetes can lower their chance of developing long-term complications like heart disease, nerve damage, kidney disease, and eye issues by maintaining their blood sugar levels within target limits.

Techniques for Monitoring Blood Sugar

Fingerstick Blood Glucose Monitoring: This technique measures blood sugar levels from a little drop of blood obtained by pricking the fingertip using a blood glucose meter.

Continuous Glucose Monitoring (CGM): CGM devices employ skin-implanted sensors to track blood sugar levels constantly day and night. In addition to offering real-time glucose measurements, CGM devices can be used to spot long-term trends and patterns in blood sugar levels.

Self-Care Techniques for the Management of

Healthy Eating: Consuming a diet rich in fruits, vegetables, whole grains, lean meats, and healthy fats will assist in maintaining general health and stabilize blood sugar levels.

Frequent Exercise: Regular exercise helps lower blood sugar, increase insulin sensitivity, and lessen the risk of cardiovascular problems related to diabetes.

Stress management: Since stress can have an impact on blood sugar levels, managing diabetes may benefit from the use of stress-reduction strategies such as deep breathing, yoga, meditation, and mindfulness.

Medication Adherence: To achieve and sustain ideal blood sugar control, you must take your diabetic medications as directed by your doctor.
Frequent Check-Ups with Your Healthcare

Provider: Keep track of your diabetes management, evaluate any complications, and modify your treatment plan as necessary by scheduling regular check-ups with your healthcare provider.

Including Self-Care in Everyday Activities

Establish attainable objectives for your nutrition, exercise routine, blood sugar control, and other diabetic self-care areas. Then, monitor your development over time.

Regularity and Consistency: Creating a schedule for exercise, meal times, medication administration, and blood sugar monitoring can promote improved diabetes management.

Self-Monitoring: To maintain ideal blood sugar management, pay attention to how your body reacts to various foods, activities, medications, and stressors. Then, make adjustments as needed.

You may take charge of controlling your type 2 diabetes and enhance your general health and well-being by making self-care and blood sugar monitoring a daily routine. We'll go deeper into doable tactics and professional advice for adopting self-care routines and maximizing diabetes management in the upcoming chapters of "Thriving with Type 2."

Chapter Seven

Overcoming Obstacles and Adopting Resilience

This chapter of "Thriving with Type 2" delves into coping mechanisms and building resilience in the face of hardships for people with diabetes. Living with type 2 diabetes can come with several practical, emotional, and physical hurdles; yet, people can thrive despite the complexity of the condition if they have resilience and an optimistic outlook.

Recognizing the Obstacles

Emotional Impact: Managing the day-to-day obligations of treatment after receiving a type 2 diabetes diagnosis can cause a variety of feelings, such as stress, anxiety, fear, and frustration.

Practical Challenges: Taking care of prescription drugs, keeping an eye on blood sugar levels, following dietary guidelines, and fitting exercise into daily schedules can be difficult at times, particularly when there are other demands on one's time.

Techniques for Managing Stress and Developing Resilience

Knowledge & Education: Gaining knowledge about type 2 diabetes, how to manage it, and what services are out there will help you take charge of your health and make decisions about your care.

Positive Thinking: Stress can be decreased and general well-being can be enhanced by adopting a positive outlook and viewing obstacles as chances for development and education.

Seeking Support: For direction, inspiration, and helpful advice on managing diabetes and overcoming obstacles, don't be afraid to get in touch with loved ones, friends, medical professionals, and support organizations.

Self-Care Practices: Give top priority to self-care practices that support your physical, emotional, and mental health. These include regular exercise, a balanced diet, stress reduction methods, and enjoyable hobbies or pastimes.

The development of problem-solving abilities is necessary to tackle several issues associated with diabetes management, including but not limited to meal and snack planning, medication organization, and troubleshooting blood sugar swings.

Practices that Promote Calm, Presence, and Inner Strength in the Face of Adversity: Journaling, deep breathing exercises, mindfulness meditation, and other practices that promote calmness and inner strength can help you develop these qualities.

Motivational Tales of Fortitude

Personal Narratives: Discuss how you overcame obstacles and developed resilience while managing type 2 diabetes. Consider the turning points in your journey that have shaped your growth, resilience, and victories.

Community Support: Get ideas from the experiences of other members of the diabetic community who have gone through comparable struggles and come out on the other side stronger and more resilient.

Honouring Development and Advancement

Celebrate Achievements: No matter how modest, celebrate your accomplishments and the strides you've made in developing resilience and controlling your diabetes.

Focus on Growth: Accept obstacles as chances for personal development and education, and acknowledge that obstacles are an inevitable element of the path to improved health and well-being.

People with type 2 diabetes can face the challenges of the disease with grace and resolve if they develop resilience, seek support, and use coping mechanisms. The upcoming chapters of "Thriving with Type 2" will go into further detail on doable tactics and professional advice for overcoming obstacles, controlling stress, and building resilience in people with diabetes.

Chapter Eight

Getting Along in Day-to-Day Life

In this installment of "Thriving with Type 2," we delve into doable tactics and professional viewpoints on living a fulfilling life while controlling type 2 diabetes. With the correct strategy and frame of mind, integrating diabetes management into everyday routines may be easy—from managing social and professional situations to traveling, eating out, and engaging in hobbies and activities.

Workplace Wellbeing

Talk to Your Employer: Share with your employer the accommodations, breaks for taking medications or checking blood sugar, and availability of healthy food options that you require for managing your diabetes.

Handle Stress: To effectively handle workplace stress, engage in stress-reduction practices including deep breathing, mindfulness, and time management.

Keep Moving: Try to incorporate short walks, workplace stretches, or standing desk usage into your workday.
Having Dinner and Seeing People

Plan Ahead: Look over menus in advance and select healthy choices that support your diabetes control objectives before heading to social gatherings or eating out.

Be Aware of Portion Sizes: When dining out, limit your intake by splitting meals, ordering appetizers or side dishes rather than entire entrees, or requesting a takeaway container so you may keep leftovers.

Keep Hydrated: When interacting with others, choose water or other low-calorie drinks over sugary cocktails or soft drinks.

Traveling while diabetic:

Prepare Supplies: When traveling, make sure you have a sufficient supply of prescription drugs, glucose monitoring supplies, wholesome snacks, and emergency contact information.

Keep Moving: Plan your trip to include physical activity by walking around, using the stairs, or participating in outdoor pursuits like swimming or hiking.

Keep an eye on your blood sugar:
While traveling, keep a close eye on your blood sugar levels, particularly if your routine, diet, or level of activity are changing.
pursuing interests and pastimes.

Discover Diabetes-Friendly Hobbies:
Look into pastimes and pursuits that complement your objectives for managing your diabetes, such as swimming, yoga, dance, or gardening.

Stay Connected: Participate in online communities or diabetes support groups that offer chances for social interaction and support among people who have similar interests or pastimes.
Pay Attention to Your Body To maintain the best possible blood sugar

control, pay attention to how your body reacts to various activities and modify your routine as necessary.

Handling Diabetes in Emergencies

Prepare an emergency plan for diabetes patients that covers blood sugar monitoring, medication administration, emergency contacts, and what to do in the event of hypo- or hyperglycemia.

Carry identity: Keep a diabetes identity card or wear a medical alert bracelet that details your condition and emergency contact information.

Communicate with Emergency Personnel: If required, let family members, friends, and carers know how to identify and handle diabetes-related situations. You should also let them know what you need.

People with type 2 diabetes can live healthy, productive lives by managing their diabetes daily and taking proactive measures to overcome obstacles. The upcoming chapters of "Thriving with Type 2" will go into greater detail on doable tactics and professional advice for incorporating diabetes care into everyday activities and getting beyond typical obstacles to leading a healthy life with diabetes.

Chapter Nine

Gazing Ahead at the Future

In this section of "Thriving with Type 2," we look at encouraging advancements, new directions, and opportunities for diabetes treatment and control in the future. People with type 2 diabetes may anticipate creative solutions, better treatment options, and strengthened support networks to help them live well and thrive despite the difficulties of the illness as technology and research develop.

Technological developments

Continuous glucose monitoring (CGM): As technology advances, CGM accuracy, usefulness, and compatibility with other diabetes care tools and gadgets all get better.

Insulin Delivery Systems: Modern insulin delivery systems, like patch pumps, closed-loop insulin administration systems, and intelligent insulin pens, provide increased insulin administration flexibility, accuracy, and convenience.

Digital health and telemedicine: Digital health and telemedicine platforms offer easy access to medical specialists, individualized education, remote monitoring, and assistance with diabetes management.

Precision Healthcare and Personalised Med

Genetic Testing: Personalised medical methods and genetic testing allow for customized treatment regimens depending on a patient's genetic composition, illness risk factors, and responsiveness to particular drugs.

Precision Nutrition: People may tailor their food and lifestyle choices to best suit their specific nutritional needs, tastes, and health objectives thanks to advances in nutritional science and personalized nutrition counseling.

Targeted Therapies: To obtain more effective and individualized treatment outcomes, targeted therapies and precision medicine techniques seek to address the underlying processes of diabetes, such as insulin resistance, beta-cell malfunction, and inflammation.

Social Assistance and Lobbying

Diabetes Advocacy: Community-based and grassroots campaigns increase knowledge, encourage learning, and push for laws that make it easier for people with type 2 diabetes to get resources, support services, and medical care.

Peer Support Networks: People with diabetes have the opportunity to interact, share stories, trade advice, and offer mutual support in managing their condition through peer support networks, online forums, and social media platforms.

Innovation and Research

Clinical Trials: Current research studies and clinical trials explore novel therapies, interventions, and technological advancements for the management and prevention of diabetes, providing hope for better outcomes and a higher standard of living for those who have type 2 diabetes.

Regenerative medicine: Methods like beta-cell replacement treatment and stem cell therapy show promise in treating type 2 diabetes and restoring pancreatic function.

Self-determination and Adaptability

Self-management and Empowerment: People with type 2 diabetes feel more resilient, autonomous, and self-efficacious when they are given the tools they need to actively participate in their treatment, make educated decisions, and speak up for themselves.

The cultivation of a positive mentality, resilience, and emotional well-being through mindfulness practices, stress management strategies, and self-care activities has been shown to improve overall quality of life and support people in thriving despite the difficulties associated with diabetes.

People with type 2 diabetes must stay aware, proactive, and optimistic about the prospects for better care, support networks, and quality of life as we look to the future of diabetes management and care. People with type 2 diabetes can anticipate a better and healthier future by being involved, speaking up for their needs, and seizing opportunities for empowerment and innovation. Let's continue to encourage one another, acknowledge accomplishments, and work towards a day when all people with diabetes can live healthy, fulfilling lives.

www.ingramcontent.com/pod-product-compliance
Lightning Source LLC
Chambersburg PA
CBHW070720260726

48660CB00007B/2664